Natural Testos

A Guide to Skyroc and Transfor.

By Sean Ward

Adherence to all applicable laws and regulations, including international, federal, state, and local governing professional licensing, business practices, advertising, and all other aspects of doing business in the US, Canada, or any other jurisdiction is the sole responsibility of the purchaser or reader.

Neither the author nor the publisher assumes any responsibility or liability whatsoever on the behalf of the purchaser or reader of these materials.

Any received slight of any individual or organization is purely unintentional.

Table of Contents

Introduction

Chapter 1. Testosterone and the Human Body

What is Testosterone?

The Signs and Causes of Low Testosterone

Chapter 2. Benefits of Increasing Testosterone

Symptoms of High Testosterone

Chapter 3. Foods to Skyrocket your Testosterone

Chapter 4. Testosterone Boosting Exercise

Chapter 5. Testosterone Killers to Avoid

Conclusion

Introduction

First and foremost I want to thank you for reading the book, "Natural Testosterone Boosting".

In this book you will learn how to naturally increase your testosterone levels and maintain these levels through eating right, exercising and avoiding things that I like to call the enemies of testosterone. All will be revealed.

Any man who takes action in his life and utilizes some of the natural ways to boost testosterone is going to realize that this hormone is not just a hormone that improves our sex life. Increasing your testosterone has many more benefits and if you can follow the tips and advice in this book you too will feel these positive changes in your body and mind.

It is my goal through the pages of this book to educate you on what testosterone is, why we need it and the benefits this hormone brings to us, what it actually does and how you can regain it when it is gone or at its lowest levels. The goal of this book is for you to become the best that you can be in your life and I can wholeheartedly say that increasing testosterone is going to help you achieve this. This book is not a medical journal and I am not offering you medical advice. The content in this book is for educational purposes only and you should consult with a licensed physician before taking any actions to increase your testosterone levels.

Thanks again for reading this book, I hope you enjoy it!

Chapter 1 – Testosterone and the Human Body

When many of us hear the term testosterone we usually associate it with the sex drive hormone. In fact for the past few decades there has been a stigma and a shame associated with the term and visions of fighting and violence spring to mind for some people, but what a lot of people don't realize is that having good levels of testosterone will make a man healthier, more productive, calm and successful.

In this book we will cover the many reasons we want to maintain high levels of testosterone, the things that will cause us to have lower levels and what we can naturally do to keep our testosterone flowing.

What is Testosterone?

Testosterone is a hormone produced by the body through the sex organs. This hormone is present in both men and women but is the primary hormone in men. The prominent sex hormone in women is estrogen.

When testosterone travels through the body it has a major effect on the sexual characteristics of men. It is in our body all of our lives but starts to really get things rolling when we hit puberty. When testosterone is produced it helps with the growth of the male sex organs, the penis and scrotum.

When men begin to produce testosterone on a regular basis they become fertile starting to produce viable sperm that are capable of producing offspring. Besides sexual aspects of testosterone it is also responsible for strengthening our vocal cords, the dreaded cracking and voice changes we experience as teens, starts to produce body hair all over our body requiring us to start shaving.

When our bodies start to produce testosterone we also begin to fluxgate our metabolism. When we start producing this hormone we are able to control our fat distribution which is another great benefit of increased testosterone. In a nutshell this means that men will start to look lean and trim a prime specimen to attract a mate.

Later Years

When we are in our later teens and early twenties we seem to have the world at our fingertips. We look good, feel good and have a sex drive that just won't quit. The problem is that this feeling of greatness doesn't last for long. In fact many men start to lose testosterone when they hit thirty of forty years of age. With the increase in chemicals, additives and preservatives that we come in contact with on a daily basis a pattern or earlier decline is becoming apparent but make no mistake this does not have to happen and if you follow some proven steps you can keep your testosterone flowing even as you get older.

The Signs and Causes of Low Testosterone

As we get older it is natural that our bodies will start to produce less testosterone than when we were in our 20s but armed with the correct knowledge when can lessen this and hold on to our precious T. The problem that many of us in our society are experiencing is the lower levels of testosterone in men who are in the prime testosterone producing years of their lives.

When a male produces less testosterone they begin to feel sluggish and less of a person with little to no motivation to take on life. As a result many men are looking for the quick fix solution that seems to be the rage in our culture. The truth is if you add in artificial testosterone into your body without understanding why you are losing it in the first place you are doing more harm than good.

In this section we will address the main causes of low testosterone and give you a few options to address the problem naturally without resorting to artificial measures.

Before proceeding through this chapter I want to make it clear that I am not a doctor nor am I giving you a medical diagnosis to your specific condition. You need to consult a doctor that specializes in low testosterone conditions for a final diagnosis. This is for educational purposes only.

Being Overweight

When we are overweight we first of all make our bodies work harder. When we work harder our bodies begin to change on a chemical level which affects all of our systems in a negative way, but that's not all.

One of the most devastating ways being overweight lowers testosterone is that an enzyme called aromatase which is found in body fat will become extremely active in your body when you are overweight, and this enzyme is responsible for converting your precious testosterone into estrogen which no man wants so we really need to lose body fat if we want to increase testosterone.

You see, what happens when you pack on too much body fat is that your testosterone will decline from the aromatase enzyme converting it into estrogen, and one of the most important ways to lose body fat is for us to have optimum levels of testosterone so we have to stop this dangerous cycle and start to lose the pounds as soon as we can.

Another way being overweight is bad is that when we are overweight we begin to change the foods in our body into fat quicker than we can burn them for energy. One of the main producing factors for testosterone is cholesterol. Now before I get too far ahead of myself there are two types of cholesterol. There is the good cholesterol that comes from farm raised animals and dairies that don't use harsh chemicals on their crops. And then there is the bad cholesterol when we eat fatty meats and foods high in sugars and starches.

The first thing that you want to do if you are overweight is to talk to your doctor or use a quality saliva test kit to see how your body is producing testosterone and what it is doing with the foods that you are eating. Many of us struggle with weight issues all of our lives and as we get older the conditions only get worse so let's take action and move in a positive direction.

Prolonged Stress and Stressful Situations on the Body

If there is one enemy to our testosterone we want to avoid it is stress, it is not an exaggeration to say that if we can lower stress we won't only be taking steps to increase testosterone but every part of our life will change for the better. When we become stressed our bodies begin to produce a chemical called cortisol. When cortisol enters our bodies it begins to wear us down. It begins to eat away at our muscle as well as vigorously attacks our testosterone levels.

Now there is a natural enzyme that our bodies produce called 11ßHSD-1. This enzyme is usually enough to protect your testosterone but with prolonged exposure to stress even this enzyme can't win the war. When this enzyme breaks down so does your testosterone levels.

When you find yourself in a prolonged stressful situation it is vital to your health and wellbeing to take a step back, remove yourself from the situation and recoup. There are many ways to avoid stress and here are a few.

- Learn to train smart, give the body a strong stimulus and push yourself but without doing so much that you are exhausted the day after or you will be kissing goodbye to your testosterone. Monitor yourself after training to know how much is right for you.
- Use an adaptogen herb like Ashwagandha that helps to lower stress and allows the body to deal with stressful situations better.
- Make sure you have some time each day that you can relax whether that is listening to some relaxing music, meditation, yoga etc, this will help your body to charge its energy back.
- Learn to laugh more and see that life can be humorous if we look for it.

If you fail to find ways to lower stress then you will continue to decrease your testosterone levels as well as do additional damage.

Alcohol

Now I know what most of you are saying, when you drink alcohol you get a little frisky and your inhibitions are lowered and most people want to go and have sex. Well this might be true but it really doesn't have anything to do with the production or lack of for testosterone.

When you consume alcohol you are shutting off nerve impulses to the brain. When these impulses are shut down so is the production of testosterone.

Other factors you will want to consider when drinking excessive amounts of alcohol is that your liver can no longer metabolize estrogen when you are forcing its primary function to be filtering out your alcohol. As you know estrogen is the opposite hormone to testosterone and when you have too much estrogen your body will refuse point blank to produce testosterone.

When you drink on a regular basis or partake on binge drinking with your buddies your body will begin to lower the activity of the enzyme known as P45. This enzyme is needed by the body for healthy testosterone production.

When we drink alcohol we usually do it to relax and make ourselves feel better. Well this is only a temporary fix and with the continuation of excessive drinking our body enters a stressful state and begins to produce cortisol which you already have learned is a big enemy of testosterone.

And the final major reason to reframe from drinking alcohol is that when you consume enough alcohol your body begins to produce a toxin known as acetylaldehyde that has been proven to lower testosterone levels. Now although alcohol does lower testosterone when it is consumed in moderation (1 or 2 drinks) this will not have such a major impact on your testosterone levels.

So to sum it up, alcohol does lower testosterone but if you are someone who can be moderate every now and again you have nothing to worry about, however if you are someone who finds it hard to be moderate it might be time to have a break to feel the positive impact this can have on your life and hormones.

Depression

Depression is becoming a serious problem in the world today. For many of us there is a hormone imbalance caused in the brain that puts us in a depressed state. Now there are medications and therapies that many people are given to help with their depression but this has little effect on the decrease in testosterone levels in our bodies.

When we are depressed we begin to send that dreaded cortisol enzyme throughout our bodies. This enzyme interacts with our bodies and as a result cause havoc with our testosterone.

There is clearly a link between depression and testosterone meaning that when we are depressed the physical changes that occur like higher cortisol have a knock on effect that leads to lowering testosterone and similarly when you have higher levels of testosterone you just naturally feel more upbeat and calm, this has been shown to be true when monitoring men's mood improvements who have undergone testosterone replacement therapy which is not something I recommend but shows the power of testosterone to improve mood, from my own experience I know how high levels of testosterone can improve mood significantly.

Having said all that, to deal with depression the right way you will need to go and get diagnosed. This diagnosis process will require you to see a medical doctor as well as a psychologist. When it comes to depression many people are afraid to see a doctor. This should not be a factor. If you feel that you are not yourself only ignoring the situation will only make it worse.

When it comes to depression this can be due to many factors such as a personal loss which can be a temporary condition or it can be due to an imbalance in your brain chemistry. So get yourself checked out before any depression tendencies get worse.

Lack of Sleep

Our bodies need rest. As humans we need at least eight hours of uninterrupted sleep so that we can let our minds rest. When we do not get enough sleep our minds, physical actions and overall health begin to fail. Our bodies begin to shut down and as a result our testosterone levels decrease as well.

When it comes to sleep finding the time to sleep is critical. If you don't get enough sleep at night you need to find time to catch a quick ten minute nap here and there even though this isn't the best solution it is better to get a nap than fight through sleep.

When it comes to the factors that cause us to lose testosterone these are only a few. Our diets, vitamins, prescription medications, exercise and overall health are also major factors. When it comes to testosterone it is vital that we keep a well balanced system so that what testosterone we have is being used and produced at its optimal levels.

Chapter 2 - Benefits of Increasing Testosterone

When we think of increasing our testosterone levels the main benefit that comes to mind is our increased sexual appetite. We feel that the testosterone that flows through our bodies is the super power fluid that helps us perform at our top performance levels in every area of life whether that is in the sports field or in the office.

Besides this benefit there are many other reasons why you would want to increase your testosterone levels. Some of them will be for physical appearance while others will be towards energy. No matter which reason you decide to increase these levels going through the process is a good idea.

Lean Muscle Mass

The first reason is to increase your lean muscle mass. When we get older we begin to lose that fine definition that we had when we were younger. This condition is usually contributed to the lifestyle and foods that we eat later in life. If you increase your testosterone levels you are allowing your body to manage your muscles better. After increasing testosterone for a period of time you will see this transformation in muscle mass taking place in front of your eyes.

Increased Bone Health

When you increase your testosterone levels you are helping your body manage calcium better. When you can manage calcium you are helping increasing your bone health which is very important as we get older.

Improved Mood

When you increase testosterone our bodies look better and even feel better. When these factors come into play we begin to improve our mood and outlook on life. When we increase our testosterone levels we feel much younger and that is always a plus.

Another benefit to increasing your testosterone is to help with depression and unhealthy thoughts. When you increase your testosterone the effects of depression are lessoned or are gone as well as the need for medications may become lessened. Don't stop taking any prescribed medications if you take testosterone without consulting your doctor.

Increasing your Metabolism

When you increase your testosterone levels you are helping to increase your metabolism. When you have a higher metabolism you will be able to eat more food and burn it for energy faster. When this occurs your body doesn't store fat cells like you would if your testosterone and metabolism levels were lower. As discussed above when we burn more fat this leads to more testosterone in the body which again leads to more fat burn.

More attractive to the opposite sex

When you have increased testosterone in your body to high levels this hidden scent becomes more active to women's senses. When this occurs women will flock to you like never before.

When women look at someone with high testosterone it first hits them on a visual cue. This is usually by the increased muscle tone of the male, the glistening of sweat or shine on their skin or just an overall presence that the male will project. The second thing a woman will pick up on is the calmness of this man as when testosterone is high there is a natural calmness and poise that can be witnessed.

When a male is low on testosterone they will not have this glow. Their personal confidence will waiver and the outward projection to the opposite sex will not be as pronounced.

When it comes to attracting a mate testosterone is usually the first thing a woman picks up on. The rest will be up to you and your presence and attitude.

Benefits Recap

These benefits are only a small list of what happens when dealing with testosterone. When you increase your testosterone levels you are taking a dip into the fountain of youth. Just think back to when you were younger and your testosterone levels were at their peak levels. Remember all of the possibilities that awaited you. Now I am not saying that you will be the He-Man you were in your prime but you will receive massive benefits from the increase. The levels and your results will vary on many factors. Also, consult your doctor before engaging in any testosterone boosting activities.

Symptoms of High Testosterone

There are times in life when our bodies will produce more testosterone than normal. When we get older this may be a desirable trait but when we are younger this condition may not be desired as much.

Some reasons our bodies will produce too much testosterone are premature puberty, increased male sexual characteristics in women and much more. In this section I am going to go through some of the most common reasons for increased testosterone and why it is not desirable.

Hyperthyroidism

Hyperthyroidism is a condition in which the thyroid begins to act up and begins producing more testosterone in the body. If this condition continues you can begin to experience a lot of different physical conditions. These conditions can be as mild as hot and cold flashes to cancer. If you are experiencing issues with your thyroid you will want to consult your doctor to see what medications and other treatments can be applied.

Anabolic Steroids

When taking anabolic steroids you are taking a huge dose of artificial steroids. When you take these steroids you are increasing muscle mass, endurance and many other factors that are popular for athletes.

The most common group of individuals to take anabolic steroids are athletes. The most common area are runners, weight lifters, boxers and other who require strength and endurance to stay on top.

When you take these steroids for an increased period of time you will begin to affect other areas of your body such as shrinking of your sexual parts, loss of sex drive and other factors that naturally producing testosterone gives us.

Adrenal Gland Tumors

The adrenal gland is a yellowish gland that sits above the liver and helps to regulate many bodily functions. When this gland malfunctions there are very little outward signs. If symptoms do appear they will manifest themselves as a lump on the abdomen.

Precocious Puberty

Testosterone becomes apparent when we enter puberty. Puberty is the state in the lifecycle when we begin to take on the sexual characteristics that we will use in our later years. These characteristics are deepening of the voice, facial and other body hair, the production of sperm as well as the increased desire for sexual interaction with the opposite sex.

When a child enters into puberty at an early age they will begin to produce these characteristics. In general this condition will reverse itself and those who are affected will go on to live normal adult lives but in some cases those who are affected will not reach their mature height since their bones will stop growing due to the condition.

If this condition occurs in girls they may fail to produce their full sexual maturity or have other issues with conception later in life. For women they may also have more body hair and other medical conditions which like in men should reverse themselves.

Illegal Drug Use

We talked about steroids earlier and that is the main drug that will cause the production of excess testosterone but other drugs may also cause issues with the body that can cause havoc with testosterone. Any time you use illegal drugs you are taking a chance on doing lifelong damage to your body. These damages can cause problems with the organs that regulate the production of testosterone.

Cancer

There are several cancers that when introduced to the body will cause psychical changes. In many cases cancers can be treated and maintained with drugs, radiation and other therapies. Since these are foreign bodies in our body there is a high risk factor that they will increase the production of testosterone in the body.

Symptoms of High Testosterone Conclusion.

When it comes to the production of higher than normal levels of testosterone in our bodies there is a common factor that can be observed. This condition is usually due to the introduction of foreign drugs into our system or a medical condition with another organ such as the thyroid working in a manner it was not supposed to.

If any of these are a factor it is highly recommended that you stop taking these foreign drugs and seek natural methods that will bring you great benefits without any consequences at all.

Chapter 3 – Foods to Skyrocket your Testosterone

There is an old saying, you are what you eat. And in the case of testosterone boosting foods you are what you don't eat. When it comes to eating we have fallen into the grab and go, eat what you can society. It appears that we spend more time trying to figure out who is doing what on Facebook than spending the time to eat a healthy diet that can skyrocket our testosterone and life in general.

When we get older our bodies take in foods differently than we did when we were younger. When we were younger we could eat anything and not gain weight, have plenty of energy and could stay up till the cows came home. Now that we are older we have trouble getting up in the morning, eat a chocolate bar and gain 30 pounds and find ourselves in bed by nine o'clock.

Well if this is a pattern that you are in then you need to take a step back and look at the foods that you are eating, how they make you feel after you eat them and what foods you can substitute for these energy killers.

In this chapter I am going to go through the top 20 super foods that you need to add to your diet in order to increase your energy as well as your testosterone levels. It is a good idea to add these foods into your diet on a regular basis.

Honey

Honey is the nectar of the gods. Made from bees this food is great as a natural sweetener. When baking or even when you drink your coffee and tea. You might also want to consider putting a few drops of honey into your baked goods and other foods to help cut down on the artificial sweeteners as well as the grain sugars we crave. This will also help to increase your testosterone levels by giving you a dose of boron which is a potent ingredient for increasing testosterone levels.

Cabbage

Cabbage is a great source of indol-3-carbonol which lowers the levels of estrogen in the body making testosterone more effective. Also broccoli and cauliflower will have the same positive benefit of lowering estrogen which is something we need to keep low in the body.

Asparagus

Asparagus is one of the world's super foods that should be added to everyone's diet. When you eat asparagus you are adding folic acids, potassium and Vitamins E to your diet. When these are processed by the body they help to increase your testosterone levels naturally.

Garlic

Garlic is one of the main foods that I personally use in all of my cooking. When you consume garlic you are helping to reduce the stress levels of the body in a natural way. When you reduce stress you are reducing one of the main causes for low testosterone levels.

Eggs

Eggs are so vital to testosterone production. When you consume eggs you are consuming potassium, vitamins, omaga-3 fatty acids, saturated fats which all form the building block for testosterone. If you eat eggs in the morning, afternoon or at dinner you are giving your body what it needs to help produce testosterone.

Bananas

Bananas are a great source for potassium as well as bromelain which is an enzyme that is a key player in testosterone production. If you are not a fan of bananas you can try pineapple. If you like both blend them together into an awesome smoothie.

Watermelon

Watermelon has been coined the all natural Viagra. When you eat watermelon you are consuming citrulline which is an amino acid that when broken down in the body produces arginine which helps increase blood flow which helps with testosterone in the body.

Ginseng

Ginseng is great for the human body. Studies have shown that taking ginseng helps men with erectile dysfunction to have stronger erections and anytime we have an erection testosterone rises.

Almonds

Almonds contain zinc which has been shown to increase testosterone as well as the overall sex drive for men and women. Take a handful of almonds an hour before engaging in sex and the experience will be much more enjoyable. Trust me on this one.

Oysters

Now I know many of you have probably heard that raw oysters are a great sex enhancer. Well you are right. Oysters have been found to contain the highest levels of zinc in any food on the planet. When you consume zinc you are helping to increase your testosterone levels as well as the overall effectiveness of your sexual activity.

Oats

Oats contain a lot of zinc. This zinc is a natural booster of testosterone. Eating oats in the morning will not only give you a warm feeling in your body on those cold winter mornings but will give you the extra boost of testosterone if you decide to stay at home and snuggle under the covers with someone.

Citrus Fruits

Citrus fruits are a great source of vitamin A. When you consume citrus fruits you are lowering estrogen levels as well as helping to produce more testosterone. Some of the more popular citrus fruits are grapefruits, Kumquats, lemons, limes, oranges and Tangelo just to name a few.

Spinach

Well we all know what happens when Popeye cracked open a can of spinach. He grew all big and strong, filling his body with testosterone which allowed him to beat his enemies wherever they appeared. Well you might not be getting super strength from spinach but you are increasing your testosterone levels. When you eat spinach you are consuming magnesium, vitamins C and E which are key components to increasing your testosterone levels.

Grapes

Grapes are great fun to eat as a snack. You want to eat red grapes though since they have been found to help increase your testosterone levels the most. The way they do this is the skins have been found to contain resveratrol that is a proven and potent aromatase inhibitor, this allows more free testosterone in the body. When you eat grapes you are also helping to increase the overall health and number of your sperm as well.

Wild Salmon

Wild Salmon is a great fish to eat. It is a super food as well as has a high concentration of omega-3 fatty acids which has been proven to increase testosterone levels. Another benefit that has been found by Australian scientists is that wild salmon also reduces SHGB which is a hormone that attacks testosterone. So eat up and fight the testosterone levels on multiple levels.

Avocado

Avocado is another super food. This food help reduce LDL cholesterol which is a major factor in low testosterone levels. Eating avocado on a regular basis will also help increase your monounsaturated fats in the body. Other foods such as nuts and vegetable oils also help to increase these levels.

Tuna

Australian scientists have concluded in their research that eating tuna is vital to the increased levels of testosterone in the body. It has also been shown that eating tuna increases the overall health and count of sperm as well.

Pomegranate

It has been shown that drinking a glass of pomegranate juice a day helped men overcome impotence as well as increase their overall testosterone levels. When eating pomegranates you will want to protect your fingers. If you don't they will turn blood red from the pomegranate juice.

Meat

Meat has been a controversial topic for millions of years now. Well maybe not that far back but for years the debate on whether meat is good or bad for you has raged on. Well scientists in Utah have concluded that eating some meat such as steak and lamb have helped increased testosterone levels in men. It has also shown that you need to keep a healthy balance since adding too much meat to your diet may lower these levels. So I guess the battle wages on. Try this experiment for yourself. Test to see what level of meat consumption will increase your testosterone levels to the max.

Tongkat Ali

When it comes to boosting testosterone, there are certain areas that you need to make sure you are concentrating on. These areas are correct exercise, adequate rest and quality nutrition.

These three areas can have a massive impact on testosterone but along with these areas there is one herb that if taken in the correct dosage can you give you a huge boost in free testosterone.

This herb is called tongkat ali and it has the power to increase testosterone, build muscle, boost energy and significantly raise libido. Tongkat Ali is a herb that grows in the jungles of Indonesia, Malaysia and Thailand.

This herb is often known as herbal Viagra and it has been used for centuries as a powerful aphrodisiac and energy booster. The problem with Tongkat is that with this knowledge there has been a colossal amount of advertising, deception and ultimately confusion.

The confusion comes from what dosage should be taken for increasing testosterone and also how to find pure forms of Tongkat Ali. The correct dosage for Tongkat to elicit a testosterone boosting response is 1:200 and this also needs to be cycled to avoid the body building a tolerance to it.

Now when it comes to finding the pure forms of Tongkat Ali, it's important to remember that there are a lot of counterfeit and fake versions that are not FDA approved. Remember to look for Tongkat Ali that is taken from trees that are at least 10 years of age since this allows the plants and roots to mature and become potent. Also make sure that there have been tests done to check for heavy metals.

Creating your own diet

So there you have it. The top 20 foods that you need to add to your diet in order to help produce the maximum level of testosterone in the body. From this point further it is your job to incorporate these foods into what you eat.

For many of these they may be a natural addition. For others you might be thinking to yourself "ewe, I'm not going to eat that!"

If you are looking to increase your testosterone levels you need to break away from that conventional way of thinking and take action to see results. Who knows, if you try it you might just see how powerful food can be.

Chapter 4 Testosterone Boosting Exercise

When it comes to increasing your testosterone levels eating healthy is only the first step. When you take in these foods you are building up your energy levels. If you don't use this energy you will be converting it into fat which is a major killer of testosterone. So in order to make the best use of this new found energy we need exercise and on a consistent basis.

Now I know that many of you are saying that you don't have time to exercise. Well I didn't say that you had to spend hour on it or start running a marathon. In fact you just need to start short and slow and build up from there.

One thing that you want to do before starting any exercise routine is to consult with your doctor. When we exercise we are putting increased strain on our bodies and we want to make sure that we exercise in the right way. Another thing that you want to do is never over exercise. One major mistake that people make is that they start to exercise and feel that if they just go a little farther or a little faster that they will see more results.

This is a myth. Our bodies are designed to work in a specific way. If we push our bodies too far they will fight back and we will become injured or overloaded with cortisol. Also another major issue that we have is doing the wrong exercises. When exercising to increase your testosterone levels you want to do specific exercises. If you do exercises that are not designed to help with your testosterone you may not be getting the desired results.

In this chapter I am going to give you a set of exercises that you can do to increase your overall testosterone levels. It is highly recommended that you do these at a slow pace and never do more than you can handle.

Sprinting

When it comes to sprinting it has been shown that doing quick ten second sprints increased testosterone levels greatly. What you do is start at a stationary position and run for about ten seconds then stop, turn around and run back to your original position.

You are looking to perform about six to seven of these in a row before taking a break. If you are not one for running then you can supplement the sprint for a few other options. You can use a treadmill and for about ten to fifteen seconds increase your speed and then slow to a gradual pace. Another option is to use a stationary bike, gaining speed for fifteen seconds and then returning to a steady pace.

When it comes to sprinting it has been found that those who engage in this activity have increased and maintained this increase of testosterone over a long period of time.

Lift Heavy Weight

When working out you will want to add weight training to your list of exercises. When you lift weights you are helping your body produce increased levels of testosterone. The most effective way to increase your testosterone levels with weights is to lift weights at least three times a week. Anything less will not give you the desired results.

Another thing, if you don't want to lift weights then lifting heavy objects on a regular basis will also aid in the production of testosterone.

One word of caution when lifting heavy objects you want to lift them responsibly. You want to be careful not to injure yourself by lifting something wrong. It is vital that you lift with your legs and not your back. You want to reframe from lifting objects that are too heavy or are difficult to get a firm grip on.

If you do decide to lift heavy objects make sure that you do it responsibly and not to go overboard. The mindset of trying to do too much can cause problems in the long term, best way is always push yourself at just the right amount and slowly build from there whilst always monitoring energy levels the hours and days after your session. You should definitely feel tired and work hard but if you are totally beat up the day after and irritable you have only raised your stress and not your testosterone.

Take Longer Breaks

When it comes to building testosterone your body needs more time to recoup. For this you will want to wait about 60 seconds to 90 seconds before each weight lifting rep.

Now for most of you standing around waiting to rest those muscles is not an option. So to best effectively use your time at the gym you will want to engage in stretching exercises as well as other exercises for those three minutes that don't stress those muscles.

If your goal is not to increase testosterone levels through these exercises then you can continue normally. When you repeat your reps on a consistent basis with little rest, you are helping to build growth hormones as well as others but not testosterone.

Pushing your body

Now this needs to be done responsibly. If you are going to force your bodies into doing more exercise than you feel you can handle and even if you don't, you want to make sure that you have a spotter or a partner.

When you force your body you are putting a good stress on it. Unlike bad stress that decreases testosterone putting extra stress on your body through prolonged exercise increases testosterone since your body is working harder.

Before you do this make sure you have a partner or spotter at the ready so that you don't get hurt. Again injury is not a desired outcome and it only takes a second of indecision on your part or your spotter to cause injuries.

Use your Lower Body

When it comes to exercise and the increased levels of testosterone it has been found that those who focus on their legs and lower body have shown a greater increase in testosterone then those who just focused on their upper bodies.

When it comes to creating a routine that maximizes the effectiveness of testosterone production here is what you need to do.

Warm-up – It is important that you warm up your body. When you jump right into exercise you are not giving your body enough time to loosen up or to build up the blood flow needed to maximize your workout. This is why doing ten minutes of stretching and other warm up exercises produce greater and safer results.

These exercises below are perfect for increasing testosterone because they work the legs and upper body in compound movements which have been shown to elevate testosterone.

4 sets of 8 repetitions bench press, paired with 4 sets of 8 repetitions squats.

When it comes to repetition doing these exercises have been shown to produce the greatest results. When you do these exercises in sets you are adding in the confusion method which makes your body more receptive to change than doing exercises in a more scheduled fashion.

4 sets of 8 repetitions deadlifts paired with 4 sets of 8 repetitions chin ups/pull-ups.

Working your upper body is key as well as your lower body. There are many androgen receptors in the upper body and these two exercises will help to build your upper body. When you do these lifts you are increasing your blood flow as well as your testosterone levels. If you have never done these exercises before you will want to have someone show you proper form as if not done correctly there is a good chance of injury.

6 sets of maximum 10 second sprints

As stated before you need to do sprints to maximize the production of testosterone. Do these after your final group of exercises. When doing these you may want to consider getting a partner in order to tag team with. Doing exercises with someone is always more fun and motivating. This can also be performed on an exercise bike.

Cool-down

Finally you need to do cool downs. When you do cool downs you are giving your muscle groups a rest. When you give these groups a rest you are allowing your testosterone levels to increase. You don't want to do a lot of reps in a row since this will be counterproductive to testosterone production. Also, you don't want to come to a complete stop when exercising. When you cool down you are decreasing your chances for injuries.

Avoid Cardio Activity

When it comes to cardio it is counterproductive to the development of testosterone. Exercises you want to avoid are long term exercises on treadmills, exercise bikes and other activities such as running long distances. When you do cardio activity you are working on being lean and not building testosterone.

Develop an exercise routine

When exercising you want to take time to develop your workout routines so that you are on a schedule. When it comes to testosterone boosting exercises as well as exercises in general you want to be as regular as possible. So if you like to exercise in the morning then you will want to design a routine that follows a morning pattern. If you like to exercise in the afternoon or evening you want to stick to that routine as well.

One thing that you don't want to do is start exercising one day and then not exercise again for a week or two. You want to develop a routine for overall body health as well as testosterone production.

One thing to keep in mind is that if you are not familiar with the exercises above and have not practiced correct form please get advice from a personal trainer, and if you do not want to do these exercises for whatever reason you can still get great benefits from using a multi gym that has exercises such as the chest press, shoulder press, row, leg extension and leg press. These exercises will also provide the stimulus to increase testosterone if done with consistency.

Chapter 5 Testosterone Killers to Avoid

So far in this book we have talked about testosterone, why it is important to increase your testosterone and several ways to do it via eating healthy, exercising and engaging in positive activities that improve your life.

In this chapter we are going to recap a few points that we talked about before about testosterone killers. It is highly recommended that you go through this chapter and take note of what these killers are. You don't want to put in all this hard work only to do something that will kill your efforts.

Stress

Stress is the number one thing that you need to avoid in order to increase your testosterone levels. When we stress we build up chemicals in our bodies that attack our testosterone hormone. When we stress over our lives we also start to eat the wrong foods, stay inside and don't socialize with others and just do counterproductive activities that have a superficial short term effect on our bodies.

One way to reduce stress is to develop a plan for your life. Many of us stress over bills we can't pay for houses we can't afford to live in, cars we can't afford to drive and activities that just don't produce results we desire.

The first thing you need to do is develop a plan for the lifestyle you want to live. Once you have this you want to look at the activities that you participate in, the people you associate yourself with and take a good hard look at what benefits they actually give you.

If you find that these items and people are not aiding you in your ultimate goal then you need to take a step back and regroup. You need to phase out the negative people, stop eating the damaging food, start doing productive activities and even isolating yourself from people until such time you can develop your path.

When it comes to dealing with stress it is going to be a long term process and the longer you wait the harder it will be to make a change. So take it one step at a time and you will start to see results.

Become Active

Quite frankly if you just sit around, watch the television, Netflix or live your life on the Internet you are not getting the physical activity, emotional stimulation and even the sunshine that is needed to produce the increased levels of testosterone you desire.

When you become active you are performing physical activities that help with blood flow, endorphin production and other chemical reactions that help aid in testosterone production. So get out, enjoy life and the testosterone will begin to flow.

Lack of Sleep

When we don't get the sleep we need we start to put a strain on our entire body. Our reaction times slow, our attitudes become negative and a lot of other factors come into play.

When trying to get enough sleep you need to create an environment that is designed to get the best sleep possible. You want to go to bed at the same time every night so that your body becomes accustomed to a sleep pattern. You want to remove all distractions from the room such as televisions, radios, clocks, light sources and more.

When you design your room specifically for sleep you are not tempted to stay up and interact with these activities. Another thing you want to do is block all light sources. For example if you have a bathroom connected to your bedroom you don't want to have the head of the bed towards that light source. There is nothing worse than waking up because of a spouse getting up to pee in the middle of the night.

Block all windows with heavy curtains. Another annoyance is having a day off and being woken up by the sun shining in your eyes first thing in the morning.

The idea is to make sure that you get at least eight hours or uninterrupted sleep a night. When you develop a healthy sleep pattern you will just be well rounded all over.

Eating Junk Food

You don't want to eat junk food, foods which are processed or don't contain any nutritional value whatsoever. You want to avoid foods that are fried, processed, contain a lot of artificial colors, flavors and preservatives. You want to focus on fruits, vegetables and foods that are grown naturally. When you focus on foods that are all natural you are not allowing good foods into your body that may counteract your production of testosterone.

Drinking Soda

Drinking a soda here and here is okay for the soul but it is not good for the development of testosterone. If you want to boost your testosterone levels you want to stay away from soda and other carbonated beverages.

Fast Foods

When you go to McDonalds, Burger King or another one of those fast food establishments you are eating a lot of processed, greasy and salty foods. As stated earlier we live in a get it now grab and go society and going to these places may be easier and more convenient but if you are looking to increase your testosterone levels you need to avoid these places like the plague.

If you do find yourself in a position where you need to grab some fast food you will want to look and see if they have any healthy alternatives such as a salad or fruit cup. Many fast food chains are adding healthy options to their menus now so before grabbing that super sized delight you may want to see what they have on the far side of the menu.

Alcohol

After a hard day's work coming home to a nice ice cold beer might seem like an ideal option. When it comes to testosterone production you want to stay away from this sudsy goodness. When we consume alcohol we are numbing our senses and adding sugars into our body that degrade the production of these testosterone producing hormones. As discussed already alcohol can increase estrogen in the body and estrogen will rob our body of testosterone so if you can be moderate go ahead but if not then stay clear.

Ice Cream

Ice Cream may be a great summer treat but ice cream is filled with sugars and fats that are counterproductive to the production of testosterone. If you have a desire for ice cream look into getting a frozen yogurt instead. You will get the same taste without all the added testosterone killers.

Pasta

I love pasta. In fact I personally eat it once a week. Now when you eat pasta you are eating pure starch which turns into glucose. When you add glucose to your body you need to work it off quickly. If you don't the glucose will covert to fat instead of energy.

This is why you see runners load up on pasta before a run. If you are looking to boost your testosterone and enjoy a nice pasta meal you will want to eat whole wheat pasta instead of the traditional white pasta and eat this in the evening after a day of activity and exercise to replenish energy reserves.

Snacks

When it comes to snacks many of us turn to something quick and bad for us. Many popular snacks are chips, cookies, ice cream, cakes and many other choices that raise our blood sugars to a point where testosterone can't be produced. So if you have the grumbling in your tummy grab a healthy snack such as almonds, grapes or maybe a veggie tray without the dip. These snacks are good for you and will not limit the production of testosterone.

Milk

They say milk does a body good. Well in some cases it does. It has calcium which is great for your bones. Unfortunately it also has a sugar known as lactose. This lactose will prevent the development of testosterone in the body. If you want milk you will want to look at lactose free milk or almond milk.

Bad Grease and Fats

Fat like omega-3 fatty acids are essential to the production of testosterone. If we were to cut out fats all together we would be in a lot of trouble since good fats are needed for our bodies to function effectively. The problem comes in when we use bad fats or trans-fats. When eating our foods you want to avoid the bad fats as much as possible.

When frying your foods you want to use natural fats and oils such as sunflower oil, vegetable oils and other natural seed oils. You want to stay away from the bad fats whenever possible and if not possible see if there is another way to cook the food such as baking, grilling or boiling.

Testosterone Killers Conclusion

When it comes to foods and activities that are bad for the production of testosterone you want to look at it and ask yourself the question - is this food or activity good for me on the whole? If a food or activity is questionable or not good for your body in general you will want to avoid them as much as possible.

Another great way to avoid snacking on bad food that will just increase fat storage is when you have the desire to eat something not so good tell your mind that you will have this snack in 20 minutes and you will see that after 10 minutes or so your mind will have gone onto something else and the desire is not there anymore. It works for me.

Conclusion

I hope this book was able to help you to understand what testosterone is, what it does and why you need it. I also hope that the information contained in this book has been of some use to you and that you can use what I have written to better develop your lifestyle to increase the testosterone levels we all desire.

Eating healthy, exercising and living a structured lifestyle will be the best things that you can do to produce the most effective levels of testosterone in your body. If you can incorporate some of the things in this book for a period of time consistently I can guarantee you will feel better in every way.

Testosterone is so important for a man that my wish for you is that you can enjoy high levels of this precious hormone and all the benefits it can bring to you.

To learn more about how to boost testosterone in a natural way check out

www.naturally-boost-testosterone.com

21789505R00026

Printed in Great Britain
by Amazon